Eve
Is a Poem
Midlife in Rhymes

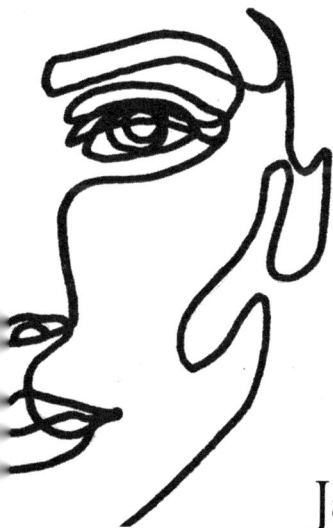

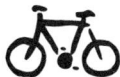

NEW ISLAND

Jan Brierton

For Alan & Cecilia

Contents

WHEN YOU'VE NOTHING
LEFT IN THE TANK...

But

The woman in me is exhausted,
The chef in me is out on strike.
The teacher in me has nothing to teach,
And the mother in me is in strife.

The housekeeper in me is dog tired,
The worker in me is off sick.
The student in me isn't listening,
And the wife in me thinks he's a dick.
(Sometimes.)

The peacemaker in me can't say sorry,
The friend in me – nothing to give.
The daughter in me pleads 'don't worry',
And the forgetter in me won't forgive.

The supporter in me has no chants left,
The juggler in me dropped the ball.
The reader in me can't finish a book,
And the caller in me missed the call.

The cleaner in me threw the towel in,
The fashionista in me looks like crap.
The beauty in me feels more like a beast,
And the gym bunny in me needs a nap.

The talker in me is gone silent,
The carer in me could care less.
The spender in me is insolvent,
And the organiser in me is a mess.

But.
The sharer in me is still sharing,
The thinker in me is still deep.
The lover in me, still has something to give,
And the dreamer in me's not asleep.

DON'T

LOSE

YOUR

SHIT

YOU'VE TOO MUCH TO DO

Hold Your Nerve

Don't lose your shit,
You've too much shit to do.
The dinner's in the oven,
And the school pickup's at two.

Don't lose your shit,
Grind your teeth and hold your nerve.
Even though you want to blow your top
And give back what they deserve.

Don't lose your shit,
Don't let them wreck your head.
Say, 'I've got a headache.'
Disappear. Take to the bed.

Don't lose your shit,
There simply isn't time.
Last night's delft is still in the sink,
And the school drop off's at nine.

Summer Hum

I'm out the back, in me fold-up chair,
I'm basking in the sun.
(I dug that Penneys boob tube out)
My soundtrack is a hum.

Not of bees in roses
or Madonna's 'Holiday',
It's mowers, drills and power tools,
Garden strimmers going all day.

Aldi did a special:
A 'High Pressure Power Hose'.
Two doors down they got one,
Their driveway fuckin' glows!

This week I'll search the middle isle,
Root through canoes and picnic rugs.
For the essential summer must have,
Noise-cancelling earplugs.

Signs of Life

Smiling
Touching
Laughing.

Holding
Talking
Grafting.

Comforting
Supporting.

Growing and cavorting.

Scowling
Shouting
Raging.

Fighting
Kicking
Ageing.

Disappointing
Offending.

Hurting and pretending.

Adult on Call

I don't want to be
The adult on call today.
I don't want to chaperone,
To the playground to play.

Or be the P.A., taking bookings
for daily play dates,
Or the driver,
Transporting them and their mates.

I don't want to referee
the sibling attacks,
Over what's on the telly,
Or, 'They ate all my snacks!'

I don't want to answer to:
'Where's my . . .'
Go find it yourself
(It's in the usual spot).

Can't *you* be on call?
While they play out the back.
Just be alert, listen out,
For screams, thumps and whacks.

I need ten, fifteen minutes,
Please, let me sit,
In silence and peace,
With a tea and biscuit.

I don't need a spa,
A massage, or a swim,
A sound bath in a room,
Where the lighting is dim.

I need a break from my shift,
We could job-share in some way?
I just can't be the adult,
On call today.

Multitask

I clean my teeth
on the loo, to save time.
In the shower I wash
and scrub off the tiles' grime.

When I'm watching Netflix,
I do the grocery shop,
And I pay the gas bill,
Waiting at the bus stop.

In a meeting at work,
I send WhatsApps and texts
about soccer and drama
and parties up in the Plex.

On my way to the kitchen,
I pick up random socks,
Throw them in the machine,
Deposit toys in the toy box.

While preparing the lunch,
I'm defrosting the dinner,
And sounding out words,
With my school spelling bee winner.

The warm steam in my face,
As I take out the dishes,
Doubles up as a facial,
It moisturises and enriches.

I've a deep conversation,
With my friend on the phone.
While I'm ironing school shirts,
We laugh and we moan

about the stresses and strains,
And the day-to-day terror,
Of choirs, multitasking
and our increased rate of error!

Hope Is in the Dark

Beneath the layers of pain,
There is hope,
On the darkest of days,
There is hope,
When you're out of your heart,
There is hope,
And as things fall apart,
There is hope.

In your wine and your nuts,
There is hope,
In the space between us,
There is hope,
In the kitchen, not dressed,
Dancing alone like a dope,
There is hope,
That is hope.

In the bad and the good
There is hope,
In the 'could', 'would' and 'should',
There is hope,
And today,
When you think, 'I can't cope',
Tomorrow is hope,
There is hope.

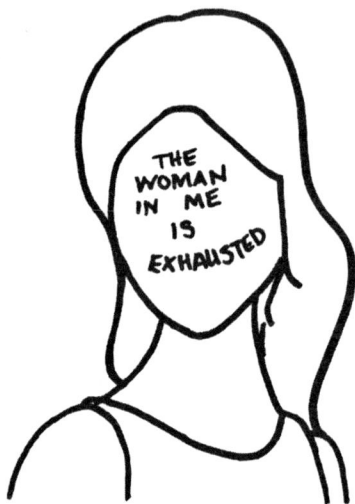

Did Somebody Say Christmas?

I forgot to move the fuckin' elf
from his hiding place behind the shelf.
I'd love a hiding place meself!
Did somebody say Christmas?

They're collecting for the school again,
For the teachers, cleaners and lollipop men,
There's a cake sale on, but I don't know when.
Did somebody say Christmas?

There's drinks for work,
I just can't miss,
We haven't met since last Christmas,
I'll go out feeling great,
I'll come home pissed.
Did somebody say Christmas?

I'll haggle with a little man,
Selling Christmas trees from a Hiace van,
To get the biggest one I can.
Did somebody say Christmas?

They'll decorate the tree their way,
Through gritted teeth – 'That's nice' – I'll say.
(When they're all in bed I'll re-display.)
Did somebody say Christmas?

I'll wrap presents that will say, 'From us',
That I struggled to get on the bus.
When he asks, 'What do you want?'
I'll say 'No fuss'.
Did somebody say Christmas?

But what I really want
is this, you see,
One night away,
Not them, just me.
So I can eat and sleep in peace,
And pee!
Did somebody say Christmas?

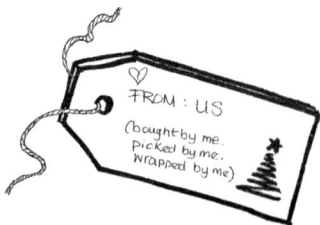

FROM : US

(bought by me.
picked by me.
wrapped by me)

NEW YEAR,
NOW YOU

Precious Thing

This year,
Be a precious thing.
Eat all the cake,
Drink the tonic and gin.

Or the wine, or the water
or the cucumber juice;
Do whatever you need
to help you produce
feelings of calm
and thoughts of *I'm good*.
Run (or fast walk)
every day round your 'hood.

You might just brush your hair,
Tie it into a bun.
Or spray on your false tan
to get milk up in Dunnes.

Tidy your house if you like,
Don't bother if not.
There's no shame in not being
a 'whatshername' swot.
Marie Kondo! Sparks joy
folding things, filling presses
and colour coordinating
all of her dresses.

Your joy might be sparked
by the gym or the sofa,
Sparkly stiletto high heels
or flat leather loafers.

You might stretch your body
on a mat in a class.
Or perhaps you find solace
in the silence at mass.

There's no 'Seven Steps to a
New Year, New You';
You're grand as you are,
You know just what to do.

Don't say 'yeah sure',
When you really mean 'no'.
And don't go to that dinner
If you don't want to go.
Close your eyes to the past,
As this new year begins.
Go easy,
Be honest,
Be *your own* precious thing.

New Year, Fuck You

Next year, let's skip January,
And have an extra June instead?
That first month's a load of shite,
It's a total wreck the head.

The dark, the cold,
The endless days,
The pressure to get fit.
You're smashed,
The party's over,
And all you want to do is sit
on the couch all day,
Devouring crisps,
Watching rubbish telly.

'New year, new you'
can fuck right off;
Embrace your lovely belly!

One Less

One less jumper to buy,
In a rushed last-minute state,
One less phone call to say,
That my day's going great.

One less plate to load up,
With stuffing and sprouts,
One less box set to sit through,
Cuddled up on the couch.

One less opponent in Scrabble,
After trifle and cake,
One less chink of a glass
of red wine over steak.

One less pint on a coaster,
On the good table inside,
One less text message to send,
After bells at midnight.

There's a space at the table,
But you're there in the tree,
In the tinsel and baubles,
the snow globes and fairies.

You're the race car in Monopoly,
The paper hats on our heads,
You're the giggles at jokes,
From the crackers at bed.

And when I open the door,
To this New Year's debut,
My memories become treasure,
That treasure is you.

WHEN MEMORIES BECOME TREASURE

Tough Love

You can't hug a photograph.
or a text that's on your phone
or a greeting card or message
or the things they used to own.

If someone means a lot to you,
Tell them today you think they're sound.
Wrap your arms around them;
They won't always be around.

Keep telling them you love them,
Even if they wreck your head,
Remind them that they're doing well.
Don't get tough, just love instead.

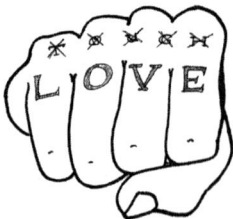

Missing

Your absence is present
at dinner and lunch,
When I catch my breath
between giggles at brunch.

When my feet touch the ground,
As I unfold from the bed,
In a fancy French restaurant,
Buttering crusty white bread.

Mouthing the words
to that song that you liked,
You said it was a 'classic'
(I thought it was shite).

Scrolling through Insta,
Typing emails,
Squeezing sliced pans
to make sure they're not stale.

And on days like this,
When the weather is pleasant,
I miss you so much,
Your absence is present.

Warm Grief

I didn't invite you here,
I didn't ask you to sit with me,
Sleep with me, eat with me.

You tap me on the shoulder,
When I lose myself in a moment
of lightness and joy,
And you remind me that you're still there.

You're ageless,
And you never grow old,
You spread over my memories of them,
Filling in the gaps.

I don't want to feel you,
But I have to feel you,
Because if I don't,
It'll mean somehow I forgot
the person that brought you to me.

And without them, all there is
is you.

There

(for Cecilia)

When I hug someone,
You'll be there.
You'll be in the mirror,
When I brush my hair,
Or carefully apply my favourite red lippie.
You'll be wrapped in my scarf,
When the weather gets nippy.

I'll see you in the trees when I walk,
You'll be in the voices of the kids when they talk.
You'll be there
while I cut carrots and veg,
And beside me
when I'm feeling on edge.

You'll look out the window
as I do the dishes,
You'll be in the candles,
When I make birthday wishes.

And when I think nobody could possibly care,
You'll do something to show me you're not gone,

You're right there.

LIFELINES

New Runners

She twists and bends
Upon the bed;
The midwife shouts,
'I see the head!

Keep going, keep going,
Just one more push.'
Student nurses stare blankly
at my wife and her bush.

Blankets unfolded,
To embrace and to wrap,
Plastic sheets are laid down
To catch any crap.

The scales are wheeled in,
prepared, ready to weigh.
She pushes and pants
and howls in dismay.

'I want you to stand,'
the midwife insists.
'Dad, we need your help,
Hold her like this.'

I hook under her arms,
Supportive and strong.
But all I can think of
In this moment is wrong.

Box fresh, brand-new leather,
Embossed with a tick.
Hurry up, have this baby.
Please,
Don't mess up my new kicks.

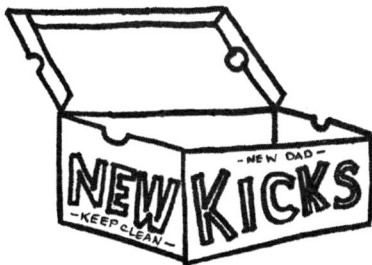

13

(for Willow)

My belly was your mattress,
I watched you twist and turn,
While you rummaged deep inside me,
A fire was lit (it was heart burn).

You stretched my skin and stole my sleep,
I felt your figure shift,
I was your wrapping paper,
You were my precious gift.

I carried you to work,
And wondered what would be your name,
My laughing was your lullaby,
My bones were your bedframe.

You left me thirteen years ago,
I'd tea and toast to celebrate,
Still today I carry you,
My heart is laden with love's weight.

These days you need me less and less,
I slowly feel redundant,
Time will pass, you'll bloom and grow,
And my love remains abundant.

School's Out

There's a banana
in that backpack,
Or an apple,
Or a pear;
A group of fruit
is hiding,
in the bag
under the stairs.

Before you settle in tonight,
Get up and root it out,
Discard half-eaten sandwiches,
Before they start to sprout.

They're lurking in the dark,
I warn you, don't forget!
Or on September 1st,
You'll unzip to find
a home-grown science project.

Lost in the Library

A woman's in the corner,
Mouthing out the As and Bs,
To toddlers and their mammies,
On the floor crouched on their knees.

At the computers, a silver surfer,
On the web since half past one,
Poking letters with his finger,
to book a week of winter sun.

Three students and their backpacks
occupy the Study Zone,
They study selfies, shared amongst their friends,
With the free Wi-Fi on their phones.

'I can't talk, I'm in the library,'
A woman hisses to her sleeve.
She opens *Zen: The Art of Living*
and breathes a sigh of calm relief.

A fella swaps a Fleetwood Mac
for a Bowie tune on vinyl,
His taste is getting better,
Last week he borrowed Spinal.

Me?
I'm lost among these shelves
of words and stories, past and present.
All life is here, between the books,
Young, old and adolescent.

When I finish reading people,
I will return to bookshelf-browser,
And if I can't find what I'm looking for,
I'll ask yer one behind the counter.

Don't Clean Today

Don't clean today,
Play cards.
Don't send emails,
Hug hard.

Instead of coffee,
Drink fizzy pop.
Sit with them on the floor,
Put away the brush and the mop.

Turn the music
all the way up to ten,
Dance on the couch,
Watch that film AGAIN!

The floor can stay mucky,
Leave the dust where it is,
It'll be there tomorrow,
Today, be with your kids.

Holy Show

The man in the dress
tells us all, 'You're a mess.'
There's only one thing we can do.

To right all of our wrongs,
We sing along with his songs,
And look adoringly on from our pew.

We stand when he stands,
Sit when he commands.
The bell rings, it acts as a cue

to kneel at our seats,
He instructs us to repeat:
'I have sinned' and 'Peace be with you'.

The basket goes round,
Coins drop, making sounds
that disturb our silent reflection.

He wipes down the gold cup,
We sit down and stand up,
And practice our best genuflection.

And all in a line,
We eat bread and drink wine.
He puts on quite the spread, don't you know.

He says, 'Go in joy,
Every girl, every boy.'
We leave with our hearts all aglow.

And if next week we're bold,
Mean or uncontrolled,
It's ok, because we all know

that on Sunday, same time,
We'll pray, 'Forgive us our crimes.'
And take our seats for the big Holy Show.

Dad

Daddy, Dad, Father, Da.
I'm so glad you got with Ma.
You're the head of the house
(She's the neck),
You enforced all the rules,
And wrote all the cheques.

Endless love and affection,
Sweets and staying up late
when Mam went out,
Every Wednesday at eight.

Never pressured, no stress,
'Work hard, do your best',
Even though I am sure
I put your patience to test.

Only now I appreciate
All that you did.
I love you, Dad.
'I love you too, kid'.

The Last Conversation
We Never Had

How was your day?
You're looking well.
Are you feeling OK?
Do you need to tell
someone about the pain you are in?
Tell me, tell me,
I'm your blister and skin.

You think I don't hear you.
But I see all your hurt.
We all feel it, we live it.
Mam goes to church
and prays every Sunday
for your safe return
from your pain, and your aching.
That one day you'll learn
to live and to love
unconditionally you.
To go easy, be gentle
after all you've been through.

Talk. I'll listen.
No solutions I'll give.
I don't have the answers.
But I want you to live.

When the numbness and dark
covers you like a quilt.
It's normal, your feelings,
of shame and of guilt.
There's much more to you
than the tablets you take
or the drink that you drown in
or mistakes that you make.

I'd tell you to work on
yourself, as you are.
To accept all your flaws,
It's not easy, it's hard.
I know, 'cos I'm learning,
To live with all mine.
Someone says, 'How are you?'
You feel shit but say, 'Fine.'

I'd say: 'Talk tomorrow.
Get some rest.
Take it easy.
I love you, my brother.'
You'd say, 'Don't be cheesy.'

Not much has changed,
Since I spoke with you last.
The kids do their sports,
Mam still goes to mass.
Dad got a new telly,
hasn't mastered his phone.
And like when you were here,
They wish you would come home.

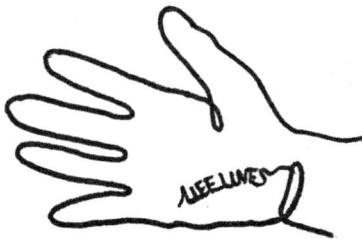

PLUS-ONES

Secret-Keepers

Secret-keepers,
Joy-sharers,
Tear-catchers,
Heart-carers.

Whinge-listeners,
Hand-holders,
Truth-tellers,
Loyalty-soldiers.

Forever-lovers,
Joke-laughers,
Mischief-makers,
Life-staffers.

Temper-tamers,
Dream-believers.
Always-there,
The secret-keepers.

Best Friend

(for Lesley)

You love me like a mother,
There's no rules, and no conditions,
Just support and ease and kindness,
You're a limited edition.

You sit with me in darkness,
When I can't see any light,
In fitting rooms, you tell the truth
when I ask, 'Is this too tight?'

You unpick my thoughts and worries,
Over coffee on the path,
In the 80s we swapped paper
that smelled like bubble bath.

You join me on the dance floor,
So I'm not dancing on my own,
Check in when I've gone quiet,
Sing happy birthday down the phone.

You're my champion,
My encourager,
You're my go-to,
My plus-one.

If love was an Olympic sport,
Then you, my friend, have won.

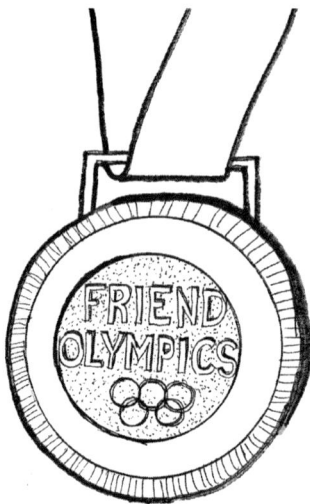

Band of Mothers

Her.
She brings mine to the park
to feed bread to the ducks,
When I've emails to send,
And my patience is fucked,
And the laundry's piled up,
'Cos my housekeeping sucks,
That's what she does for me.

Her.
She said hello
when the others did not.
Had me over for cake and tea from a pot.
Now we bond over wine,
Sometimes we even drink shots,
That's what she does for me.

Her.
She drives my young one to class birthday parties,
Drops him home full of cake,
Clutching bags filled with Smarties.
She trusts me with her two and her spare set of car keys,
That's what she does for me.

Her.
She's good with advice,
She is wise and she listens,
We talk about everything:
Music, sex, politicians,
She tells me her secrets,
I help make her decisions,
That's what she does for me.

Her.
She welcomed me in, never gave the cold shoulder,
I don't see her as much now,
But we're friendship shareholders.
And her eldest minds mine,
Now that she's getting older,
That's what she does for me.

Who knew at the gates,
That I would discover
this motley crew,
Who I love now like no other.
They care and protect,
As though they were my mother.
That's what they do for me.

Away

I'm not jealous,
How could I be?
You'll all drink and laugh,
And have chats over tea.

I've just dropped off at school,
I'll go home now to clean,
While you're in departures,
Reading glossy magazines.

Enjoy! ENJOY!
You deserve it so.
The sun, the sleep,
The time going slow.
The eating out,
The balmy breeze,
The people watching . . .

Can I come next time please?

Plus-One

He was my plus-one,
Now he's yours.
He orders drinks,
And holds open doors.
I was here before you,
Now, I'm not keeping score.
But he was my plus-one,
Now he's yours.

In the morning,
He's the first one I phone,
We talk fashion and music
and moan.
Now he's obsessed with you,
He likes the tunes that you do,
Backstreet Boys, Little Mix
and Boyzone.

He cheers you on
when you're running in Lycra.
You give him lifts
in your Nissan Micra,
He gives you clothing advice;
Honest and not always nice.
But it's gospel;
He's a fashion messiah.

Round your gaff,
He does all of the chores,
He wears earplugs,
To cut out your snores.
He changes the plugs,
Gives good guidance and hugs
when your heart's broke
and your head's feeling sore.

He was all mine
before he met you.
I don't think
we can split him in two.
Maybe half of the year,
I could just keep him here?
And you could have him
for a month or a few.

Now you'll take him
in sickness and health,
Share your life and your bed
and your wealth.
You'll kiss and share rings,
Promise only nice things,
And proclaim all of the deep love
You've felt.

He's your plus-one now,
He's not mine.
I'm not crying, I'm not!
I. AM. FINE!
I'll drink cocktails and gin,
Dance to Kylie with him,
You'll join in when they play 'Borderline'.

On the dance floor
I'll make room for you.
We'll hold hands,
And bust out some new moves,
We'll rave together, us three,
You, him and me
'Cos from today,
My plus-one's a plus-two.

DRESS YOUR SHOESIZE
NOT YOUR AGE
(I'M A 38)

Worth the Wait

You are not too old,
And it's not too late,
To dance on the table,
Or eat all of the cake.
To wave your hands in the air,
To follow the trends
and wear glitter for gigs
in a field with your friends.

To sit at a desk,
Put your hand up, ask why.
To state your opinion,
Even though you feel shy.
To apply for that new job,
To rise up the ranks
in a shop, a tech company,
One of those big fancy banks.
So go on, take a chance,
You are so worth the wait.
'Cos you're never too old
And it's never too late.

Older, Bolder

Older, bolder,
Greyer, wiser.
Slower, stronger,
Life-advisor.

Kinder, smarter,
Giver, carer.
Supporter, listener,
Life-skill sharer.

Experienced,
And looks that smoulder
With Confidence.
Older and bolder.

Sound Body

Dear body,
I didn't mean what I said
about your wobbly bits,
I love your stretch marks and scars,
And your big droopy tits.
Your round blancmange belly
And your two boiled-ham thighs.
I love the crepe paper creases,
Around each of your eyes.
I love the pimple that lodges
on your forehead for weeks.
I love the hair on your toes
and the dimples on your bum cheeks.
And though sometimes I wish,
That your legs were longer,
I'm you, you are me,
And together we're stronger.
You hold me,
You host me,
You move me around.

My body,
My gift.
Dear body,
You're sound.

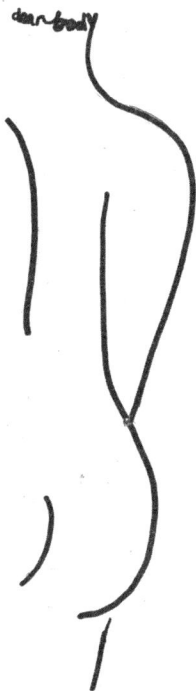

dear body

Dark Day

Feeling like a piece of piss,
Blurry eyes,
Thoughts amiss.

Fuck this.

Staying in,
Not going out,
Eating crap,
And feeling stout.

I'm not sure
that this is me;
I want to disappear,
You see.

Please,
don't look me in the eye,
I feel ashamed,
You watch me cry.

'Do yoga,'
'Breathe,'
'You'll find your bliss,'
I never used to get like this.

It hurts my brain,
To reminisce,
All I need's
A hug . . . A kiss?

Fuck this.

The Fog

A fog has descended,
It's heavy and thick,
So, I sleep and drink tea,
And hope it will pass quick.
As soon as it does,
I've no doubt I will write,
Something funny and thoughtful,
Light-hearted and bright.

For now, I'll go quiet,
I'll sigh lots,
I might weep,
I'll get up,
Even though all I want is to sleep.

I'll make dinner (again),
Like I do every day,
Put my red lipstick on,
In the hope that I may
rise and emerge!

From this desperate haze,
Return to myself
and the lightness of days.

THE FOG

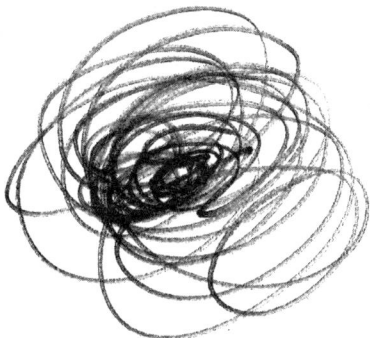

The Handbook

No one tells you your eyebrows fall out
and grow from your chin.
They don't tell you your teeth twist
and your hair gets thin.

Or that, without a bra,
Your boobs tuck into your socks.
And beyond forty-six you'll still get spots.
There's no discussing the rage –
Gritted teeth, constant 'FUCKs',
A new addition to your already complex make-up.

The fog and hot flushes,
Bigger boobs, bigger arse.
Chills, sweaty nights;
There's no midlife weather forecast.

Shrinking confidence, leaky sneezes,
Wind, a weakened ego.
Don't talk about the body-loathing or the dwindling
    libido.

And The Handbook
has no mention of the dry pain in your fanny.
You know *The* Handbook?
I'm lying. There isn't any.

Forecast

Expect an unsettled chilly night,
mixed with sweaty heat,
Followed in the morning
by a dizzy fog;
Becoming unsettled at times,

Which will clear in the afternoon,
Bringing some sunny spells
with highs of coffee and chocolate.

After which a dark rage and thunder
will become heavy and prolonged,
And will develop late into the evening.

Leaving the night clear of any intimacy,
But with scattered signs of love and support,
With tea and hugs and silence,
Pushing in from the outside.

THE ROYAL 'WE'

WHEN HE SAYS 'WE,'
HE MEANS ME...
WHEN I SAY 'SOMEONE,'
I MEAN HIM

You're Mine

After John Cooper Clarke's
'I Wanna Be Yours'

I don't wanna change you,
I sometimes wanna rearrange you.

I know I'll never fix you,
But I might just try to mix you.

I could gentrify you,
Twenty-first-century-guy you.

I'll gold plate you,
I promise I won't slate you.

When you're wrecked and feeling blue,
I'll prop you up and get you through.

I'll stand by you,
Like your man in *Grease*,
I'll electrify you.

I only want you,
When I die,
I'll probably haunt you.

Because forever, I'm yours,
And you're mine too.

She Who Comes With Her Own Things

She who comes with her own things:
Fancy clothes and diamond rings,
Modern art to hang on the wall,
Towering heels that make her stumble and fall.

Bottle and creams to keep her skin fresh,
Tanning lotions that smell and darken her flesh,
Photos of friends that you haven't met yet,
Cups, plates and saucers – all matching sets.

This was once your kingdom, your gaff, your man-shed,
But you offered to share with your heart not your head.
You didn't realise she came with all of this baggage,
You know that somehow, together you'll manage.

The clutter, the madness, the crap taste in music
(that CD of whale song is quite therapeutic).
The chores you'll share out: laundry, cleaning the loo,
They'll both be hers, you've the garden to do.

The 'big shop' each weekend, you'll stroll together
    down aisles,
You'll push the trolley, she'll buy kitchen supplies.
'Get this, it's good value,' she'll recommend.
And you'll fall in love,
All over again.

Silently You Love Me

There's loads of ways
To say 'I love you',
Without roses or chocolates,
Fancy dinners or booze.

Like bringing up my tea,
So it doesn't go cold.
Scrubbing the tiles round the bath,
To remove all the mould.

Picking your T-shirts
up off the floor.
Washing the pot from breakfast oats
(Still in the sink) at four.

Letting me sleep
while I snore and keep you awake.
Knowing what's right for dinner:
onion rings and fillet steak.

Opening the door
when I ring the bell, twice.
Complimenting my new dress;
You think it's mad but say, 'It's nice'.

Finishing your shower
so I can take a pee.
Watching 'My List' on Netflix
And sports on TV.

Flowers and chocolates,
Big grand gestures for show,
Are nice now and then.
But I want you to know:

There's no need for gifts
(OK, maybe once in a while).
I know deep down inside,
How you feel when you smile,

And ask, 'How are you,
Everything good?'
I shrug *I'm not sure.*
You wrap me up in your hug.

There's no music,
No flowers, no passionate kiss,
Your embrace needs no words,
What you're saying is this:

I Love
You.

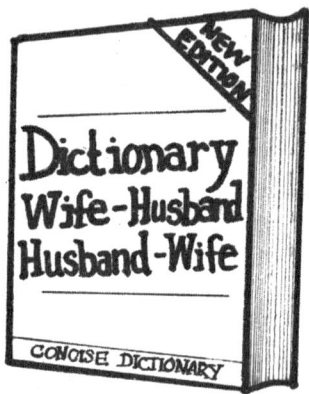

Love Is Taking Out the Bins

A hug is not the same
if you have to ask for it.
It doesn't feel as comfortable,
It's a cuddle counterfeit.

Attention, when it's begged for,
Is almost always not deserved.
It's craving recognition
to keep the ego well preserved.

Love, when it's not measured
by big gestures and nice things,
It is a cup of tea and silence,
Love is taking out the bins.

Safe and Sound

You're my safe and sound
when I've run aground.
And it's not been plain sailing,
'Cos I'm convinced I'm failing.

You're my comfort blanket,
Let me sleep when I feel frantic.
You're my painkiller,
You're my emptiness filler.

When I can't see right,
You fine-tune my sight.
When I'm lost, you're my found.
You're my safe and sound.

Tin

After ten years,
You'd think we'd be better than this,
That we'd have figured it out,
Settled into deep wedded bliss.

That we wouldn't still argue
about what I like and you don't,
About the places you'll go
and the places I won't.

That we'd be a #TeamUs,
Managing the lows and the highs,
with inspirational quotes,
Not a symphony of sighs.

'How are you?'
'I'm tired. You?'
'I'm tired too.'
At least we're tired in unison,
Together we're blue.

Together we'll make it,
We can relight the flame,
We've at least *one* thing in common:
we both feel the same.

We're still figuring out,
How to be with each other in life,
You're fluent in 'husband',
I'm still learning 'wife'.

And while we study these lessons,
I want you to know:
Ten years may have passed,
But we've forever to go.

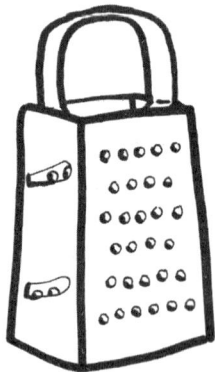

Through Love

He knows I amn't perfect,
But he treats me like I am.
He looks at me with eyes
that don't see just a knackered mam.

He quietly supports me,
Even if I lose my way,
And when he sees I'm crumbling,
He always asks, 'Are you OK?'

He doesn't see the dirty floors,
Or comment on the mess,
He doesn't say, 'Relax!'
When I'm wound up and feeling stressed.

He compliments my cooking skills,
Says it tastes just like gourmet,
And if I ask, 'Do I look good in this?'
He knows what not to say.

He talks to me in gentle tones,
When he really wants to shout,
The highs, the lows, he loves through it all,
'Cos that's what love is all about.

Romance Is in the Sink

Don't give me a card
the size of the telly.
Don't present me some trinkets,
Or a candle that's smelly.

Don't get me a rose
on its own wrapped in plastic,
Or a face cream for wrinkles,
To keep my skin elastic.

Don't buy me tech!
I don't need a watch that is smart,
I don't want chocolates in boxes
shaped like a heart.

I know that you love me,
I don't need stuff to prove it,
Just put out the bins,
And don't tell me to 'cool it'.

When I've lost the head
'cos the washing's not done,
D'ye remember we romanced,
The flirting, the fun?

Our romance these days
is in the sink filled with cups,
On the couch watching telly,
In life's downs and life's ups.

You tell me you love me,
By making me tea,
Laughing at my crap jokes,
And letting me just be me.

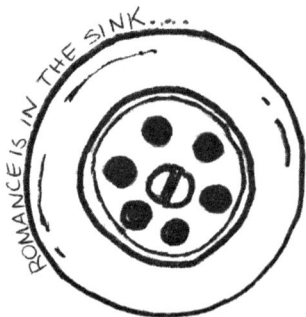

ROMANCE IS IN THE SINK....

US

(for Richard & James,
on the occasion of their wedding day)

My favourite love story is ours:
When we first met it was romance and flowers,
Now it's bills and bank loans,
Laughs and giggles, some moans,
On the couch watching Netflix for hours.

It won't always be a life full of bliss,
But today I can promise you this:
I'm yours and you're mine,
Together, we will be fine,
Let's swap rings and seal vows with a kiss.

I'll dress you up in my love like Madonna,
And choreograph a first dance if you wanna?
We'll celebrate with our tribe,
Soak up all the good vibes,
No one else throws a party like we're gonna.

It's worth all of the drama, it is!
Standing here in our suits drinking fizz,
All eyes are on us.
I'm 'Taa daaah'; you're no fuss,
But it works, we make the best his and his.

We'll grow on each other like mould,
I'll keep you warm in the damp and the cold,
Over years we'll mature,
And be each other's cure,
For the heartache of all life's untold.

There's no best before date on our passion,
No expiry, use by, there's no ration.
Just a promise of trust,
That you and me are now US,
And US never goes out of fashion.

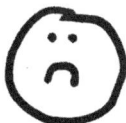

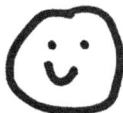

I Bet You Think This Poem Is About You

I have news:
It's not all about you.
Nobody cares about the stuff that you do:
That new thing you bought,
The new blinds that you hung,
Your haircut, your car,
How you relate to your son.

That you sometimes feel great,
On other days you feel shit.
That your leggings are tight now
and they don't really fit.
That your dishes aren't washed,
Or the house isn't hoovered.
They're too busy with theirs,
To care for your next manoeuvre.

Or that American actress
and the likeness you share.
In a good way,
I promise,
Nobody cares.

Lipstick Is My Yoga

Lipstick is my yoga,
This dress is my 5k run.
French manicures are my Pilates,
My cold sea swim is a chocolate bun.

That 'O' into the mirror,
To spread the colour everywhere,
That's my mindful moment of the day,
When *my* thoughts become so clear.

I don't need a daily mantra,
To keep my head in check.
Lipstick is my yoga,
A dance in my kitchen's my 10,000 steps.

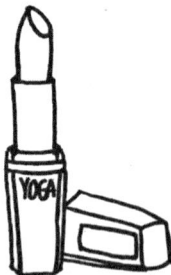

Me *Before* the Sea

You said I'd feel amazing,
You said I'd feel refreshed.
But it's been twelve hours;
I can't feel my toes
and I've only caught my breath.

Now I'm eating all the biscuits,
I'm drinking all the tea.
Anything to make me feel
like the me
before the sea.

I jumped in, feet first, no messing.
I committed heart and soul.
But you never told me,
To feel so good,
You've to get so fuckin' cold!

Next time I'll wear a wetsuit,
Get a Dry Robe to fit in.
I'll leave a flask of tea at the shelter,
With my biscuits in a tin.
I'm only getting over it.
Now you say it,
I did feel free.
But my nipples haven't been the same,
Since I jumped into the sea.

Robert Smith Eyes

(for Amy)

Always take your mascara off
before you go to bed.
It'll end up all over your pillowcase,
(The one with Egyptian thread.)
And if you're wearing lipstick –
your favourite, Ruby Woo –
Make sure, before you go to sleep,
To wipe your lips off too.

If your face took hours for you to paint
Using brushes and rouges and sponge,
Take a selfie, and share just how gorgeous you are
With the addition of all of this gunge.

We all love to dress up our faces,
Our make-up is facial couture.
But,
If you don't take it off when it's bedtime,
You'll wake up like yer man from The Cure.

Self-Esteem Repair

Our lips are getting bigger,
Our lashes getting longer,
Our hair, instantly shorter
or darker or blonder.
Our nails are long and multi-coloured,
Decorated with designs.
There's no more fuzzy frilly knickers,
These days we've clean bikini lines.
Our wardrobes, they get fuller
with clothes we never wear.
We spend all our saved up money
on this self-esteem repair.

Semi-D

At first, I learned to accept,
Now I've learned to embrace
the lumpy bits,
the stretchy skin,
the spots upon my face.

My body,
It's not quite a temple,
More like an old semi-d,
Loved, lived in, cracks inside and out,
Not perfect but just right for me.

F.O.B.I.

(Fear of Being Included)

Don't say yes,
When you really mean no.
It's OK to decline,
Change your mind or not show.

If you'd rather stay in,
In your PJs and chill,
You don't need to lie,
Or pretend that you're ill.

Your sisters, your friends,
Or the ladies who dine,
They'll text 'Oh, we miss you,'
While getting pissed drinking wine.

There'll be nights in the future,
You'll be the life and the soul,
But if this week's been tough,
And it's taken its toll,
You'll feel better at home,
No, you don't have to go.

Tell them,
'Maybe next time',
And commit to your no.

Self-Care

Become your own therapist,
Listen to yourself,
Take some time to talk to you
when you need a little help.
Tell yourself you're doing well,
It's normal how you feel.
Give yourself a rest, a break,
Jump off the hamster wheel.
Make yourself a cup of tea,
Have a slice of cake.
Take a nap, look after *you*,
Mend and soothe your ache.

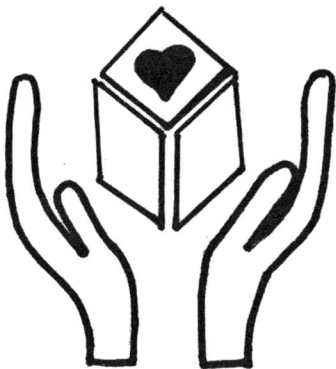

HANDLE
ME WITH CARE

Acknowledgements

I have so many thanks to give.

I must thank my agent, Faith O'Grady at Lisa Richards, along with my publishers, New Island. Thank you especially Aoife K. Walsh and Mariel Deegan for your support and collaboration.

Writing poems and having not one, but two books has been one of the greatest surprises of my life.

Massive thanks to the Band of Mothers, the Plus-Ones, the Secret-Keepers and all of the supporting cast in the poems. Thank you for the constant inspiration and encouragement. I'm grateful for the crappy days as much as the good ones, because without them there wouldn't be any light and shade in these pages.

Most of all thanks to my loves: Austin, Willow and Theo.

And finally, thank you Mam and Dad; how lucky I am to have you. x

EVERYBODY IS A POEM
First published in 2024 by
New Island Books
Glenshesk House
10 Richview Office Park
Clonskeagh
Dublin D14 V8C4
Republic of Ireland
www.newisland.ie

Print ISBN: 978-1-84840-920-0
eBook ISBN: 978-1-84840-921-7

Editing, typesetting and cover design by New Island Books
Printed by L&C Printing Group, Poland, lcprinting.eu

New Island Books is a member of Publishing Ireland.

10 9 8 7 6 5 4 3 2 1